P.M.S. ATTACKS

AND OTHER INCONVENIENCES OF LIFE

STEVE PHILLIPS

W9-AGP-880

1⊖ TEN SPEED PRESS

Copyright © 1988 by Steve Phillips.
All rights reserved. No part of this book may be reproduced in any form, except for
brief reviews, without the written permission of the publisher.

1🄯
TEN SPEED PRESS
P.O. Box 7123
Berkeley, California

Library of Congress Cataloging-in-Publication Data

Phillips, Steve, 1953-
    P.M.S. attacks and other inconveniences of life/Steve Phillips.
        p.   cm.
    ISBN 0-89815-239-9
    1. Women—Caricatures and cartoons. 2. American wit and humor.
Pictorial. I. Title: PMS attacks and other inconveniences of life.
NC1429.P57A4 1988
741.5'973—dc19

First Printing, 1988
Manufactured in the United States of America

1 2 3 4 5 — 90 89 88

Look for Steve Phillips' cartoons in these LANDMARK CALENDARS: P.M.S. Attack
wall calendar, the P.M.S. Attack engagement calendar, Mid-Life Crisis wall calendar
and Psycho Dairy Farm 16-month calendar. All available from Landmark Calendars,
P.O. Box 6105, Novato, CA 94948.

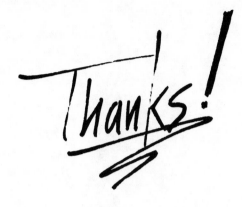

Thanks!

"Truly, without the love, guidance and influence of the following people, this Book would be a ham sandwich" Steve

Freckles of Love, Inee Hienee, Bub and Zaid, Morey Monkey, Sparticus, Radon Mcbuckets, Betty Anne Spam-cakes, Little timmy forklift, Stinky, the L.I.R.R., Paul, Joanne and Jaimie McBuckets, Bones, Stan & Marilyn "Hey lets party dude" cohen, The Landmark "Party Girls", Godzilla, "Sporty" Morty Morton, Brooklyn Melanie, Palssons Restaurant of New York and to the force that put all of these charactors here on this planet, in the same dimension, at the same time... our creator.

P.M.S. Attack #1

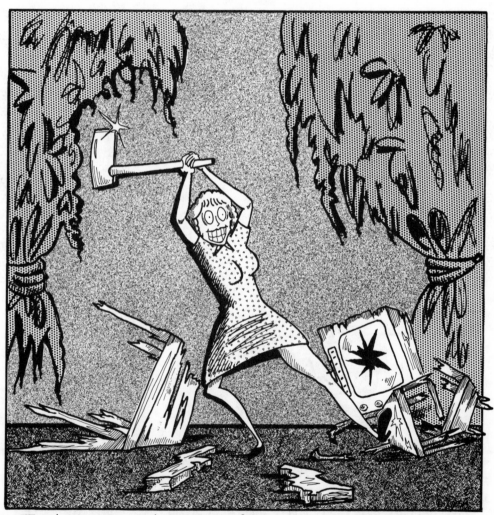

To take her mind off her Pre-Menstrual syndrome, Melinda decides to rearrange the furniture

P.M.S. Attack #2

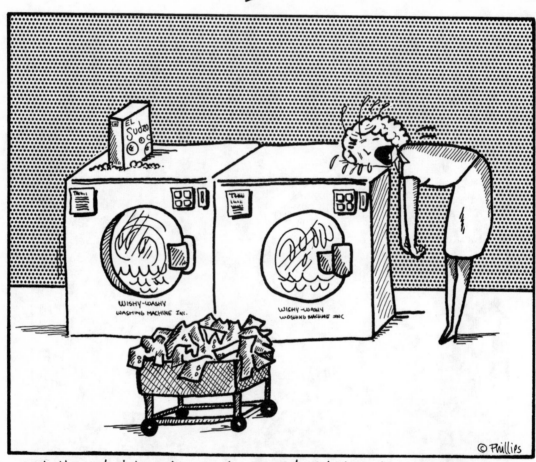

While at the laundramat, Melinda suddenly bursts into tears as she realizes the similarities between the spin cycle and her life

P.M.S. Attack #3

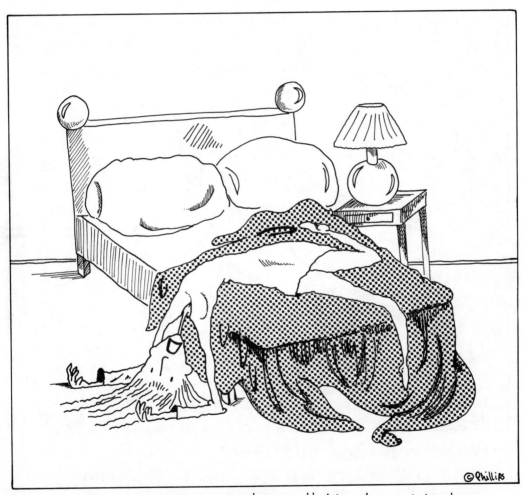

with her energy level at an all time low, Melinda
passes the time wondering how long it will take before
her body falls off the bed

P.M.S. Attack #4

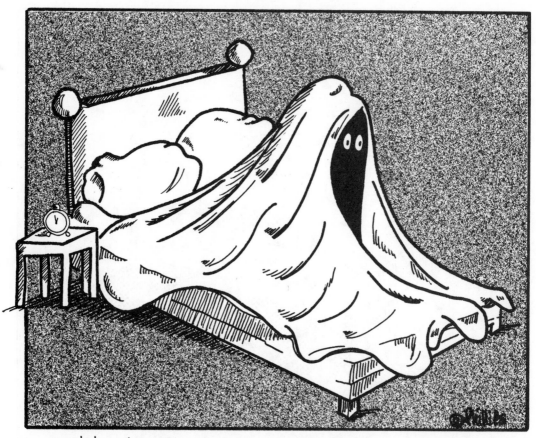

Unable to face the world, Melinda decides to spend the rest of her life under the covers

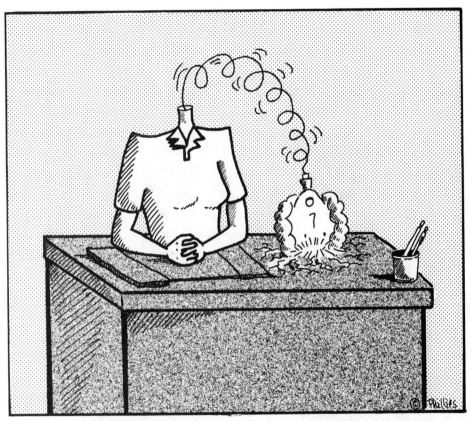

P.M.S. Attack #5

Melinda was convinced
she had it under control

P.M.S. Attack #6

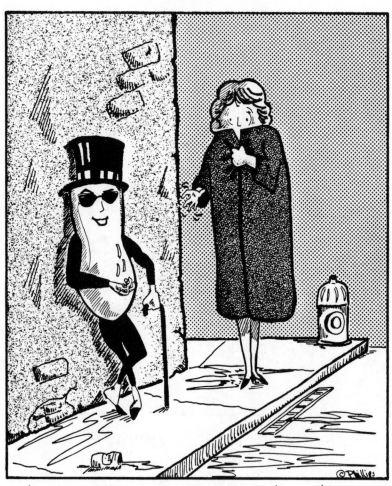

"Unable to kick her addiction to salted peanuts, Melinda visits **"THE MAN"** one more time."

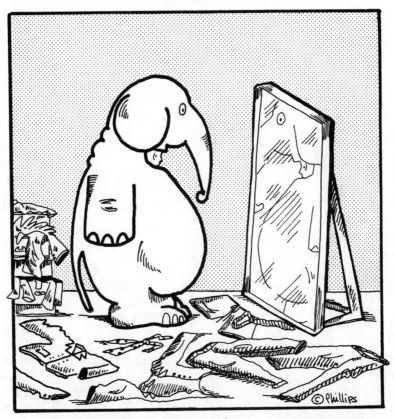

Frantically, Melinda searches in vain for the right clothes to fit her mood. SUDDENLY she remembers **THE ELEPHANT SUIT**

P.M.S. Attack #8

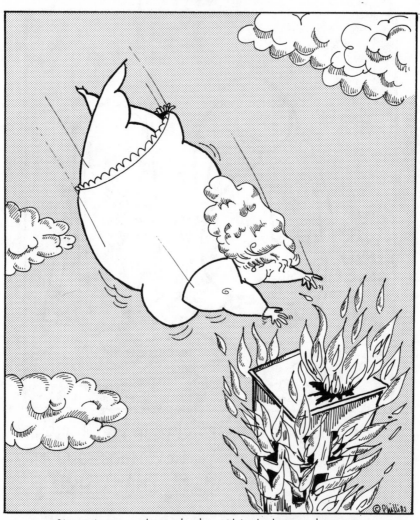

Plagued by water retention, Melinda throws herself
on a burning building and "saves the day"

P.M.S. Attack #9

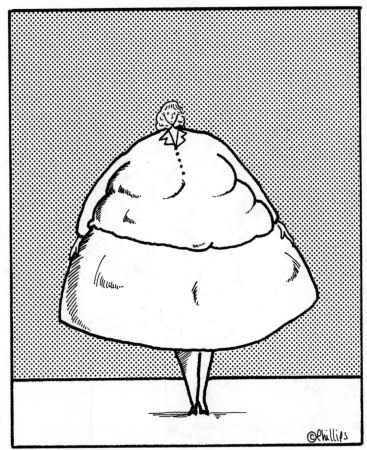

Melinda is amazed at how quickly she loses weight in her face

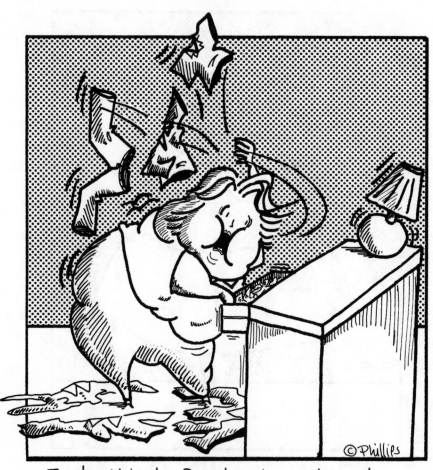

Frantic, Melinda forgets where she put...
" the FAT clothes "

©Phillips

P.M.S. Attack #11

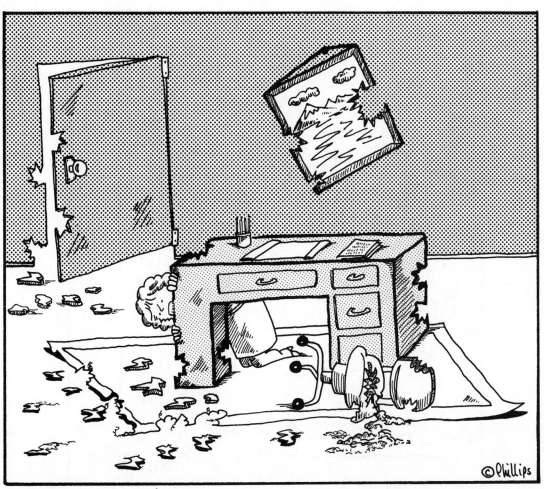

During those times of high anxiety, Melinda discovers a "sure fire" way to stop biting her nails

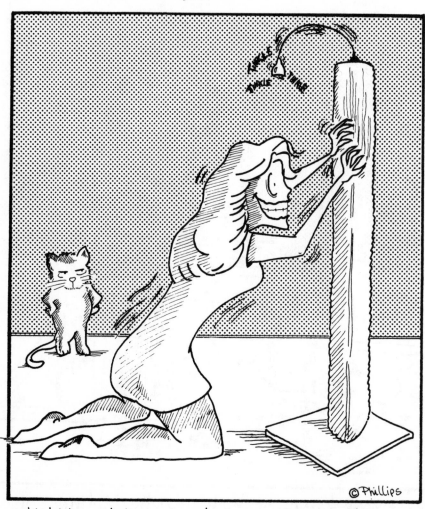

Nibbles, Melinda's cat, grows impatient as Melinda monopolizes the scratching post

P.M.S. Attack #13

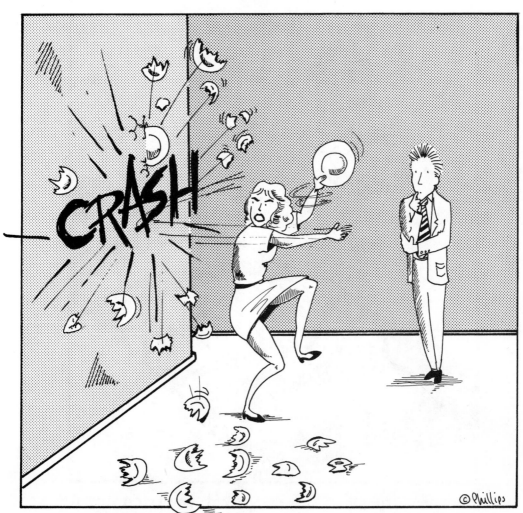

Barney wonders whether this is a good time to
tell Melinda he'd like to date other women

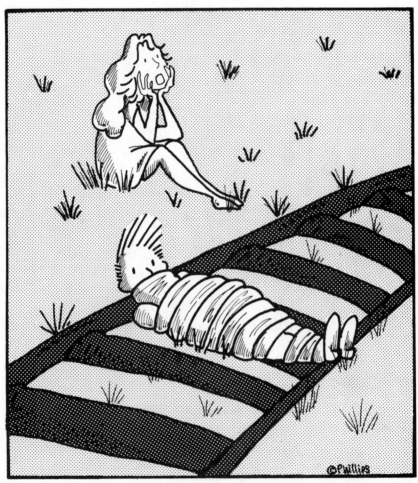

Melinda explains to Barney that her occasional bouts with stress, and irritability, shouldn't be taken personally

P.M.S. Attack #15

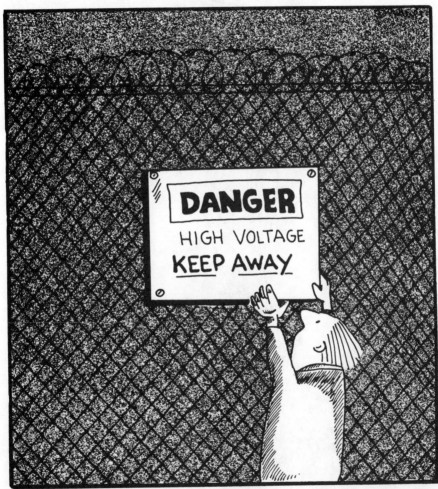

Sensitive to her needs, Barney gets Melinda
a gift for her monthly hormonal shifts

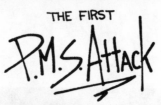

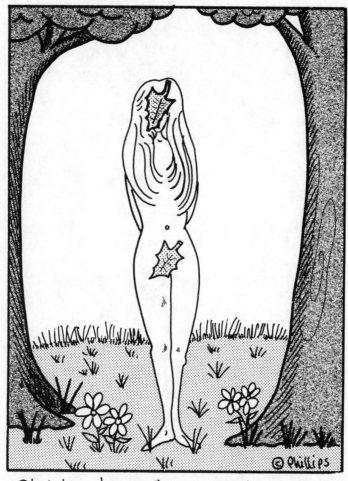

Stricken by an "UGLY MOOD" swing
EVE takes the necessary precautions

P.M.S. Attack #16

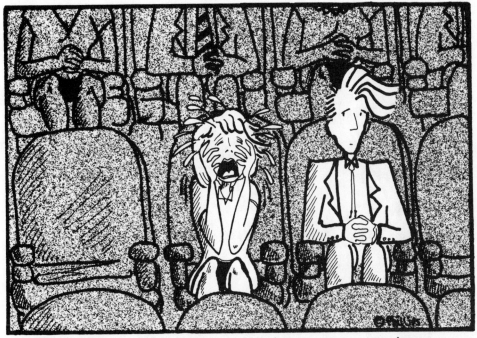

After seeing the film "Platoon" Melinda is brought to tears as she realizes that she left too small a tip at the Vietnamese restaurant

P.M.S. Attack #17

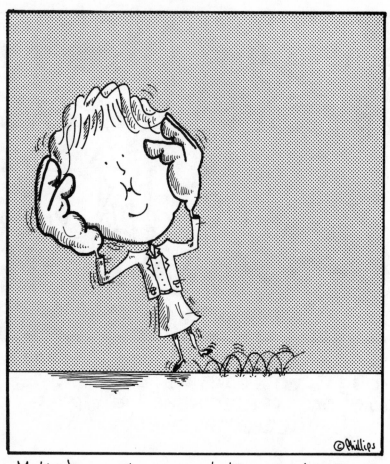

Melinda's only consolation for her
swollen hands, were that they were now
large enough to keep her swollen head
from falling to the side

P.M.S. Attack #18

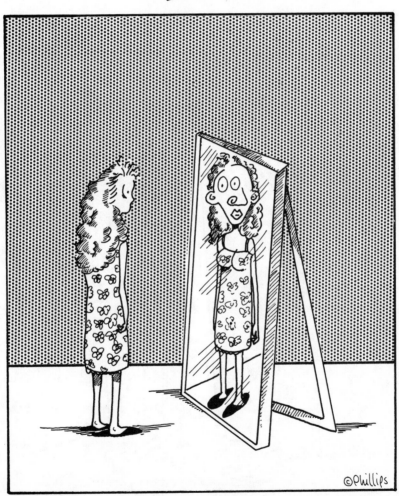

Melinda suspects that she's undergoing another "UGLY MOOD" swing

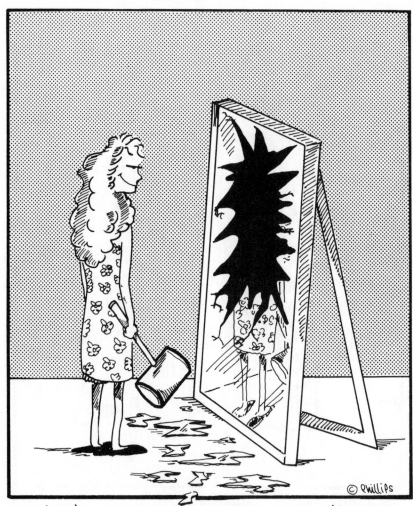

P.M.S. Attack #19

Melinda finds a way of coping with her "UGLY MOOD" swing

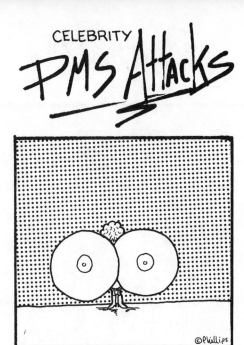

A Famous
country Western Singer

P.M.S. Attack #20

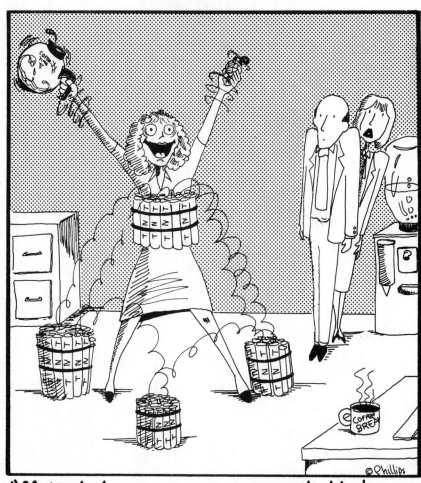

"Melinda's co-workers suspect that Melinda may have gone too far in her request for a new 'Mr. Coffee'."

CELEBRITY
PMS Attacks

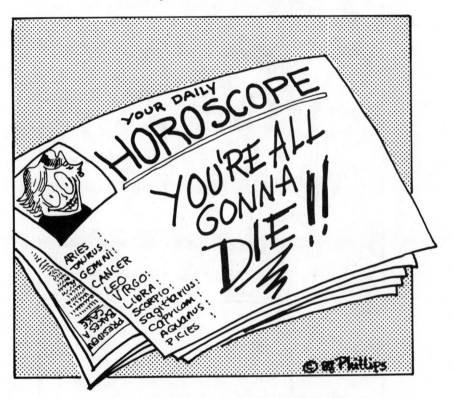

A FAMOUS ASTROLOGIST

P.M.S. Attack #21

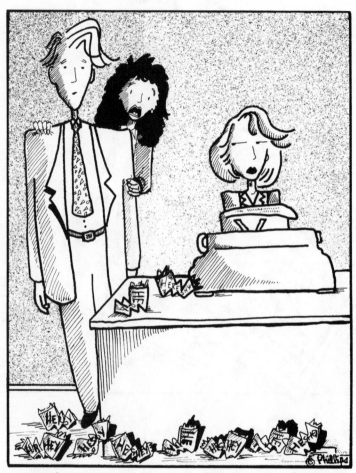

Melinda's co-workers could always tell the kind of mood she was in by the number of HERSHEY wrappers around her desk. **TODAY WAS A TEN WRAPPER DAY!**

P.M.S. Attack #22

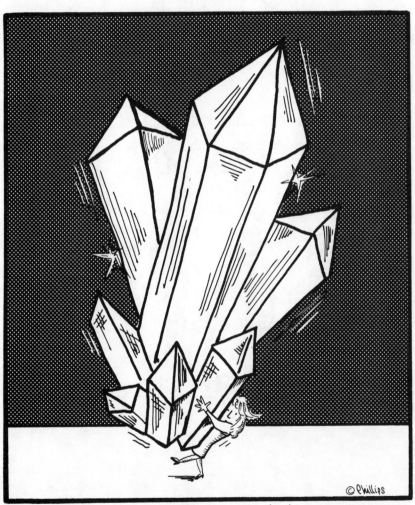

Hearing that crystals can help ease stress, Melinda purchases an appropriate one for her needs

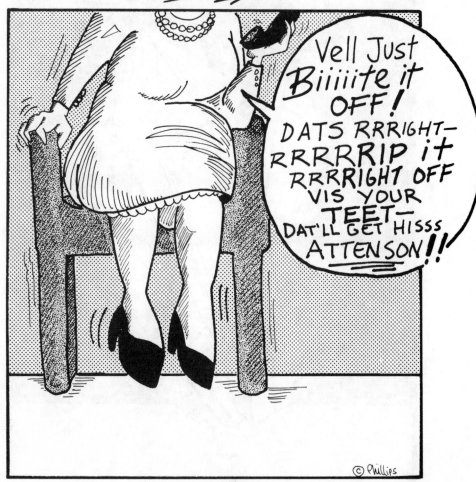

A FAMOUS
Sex Therapist

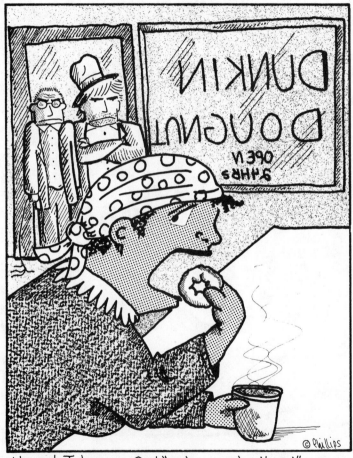

Harriet Tubmans first "underground railroad" escape was derailed when, during a severe craving for sweets, she led the slaves to a local DUNKIN DOUGHNUTS—where they were quickly apprehended

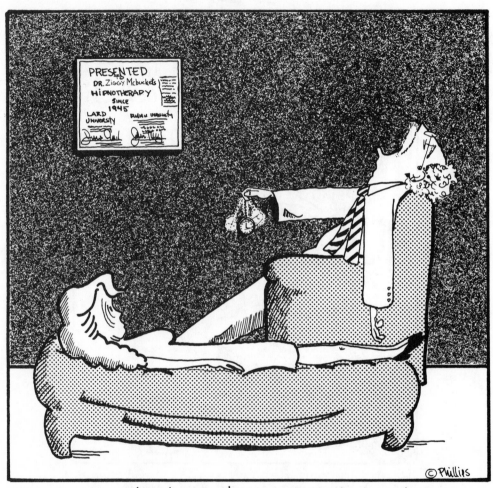

P.M.S. Attack #23

To cope with her stress Melinda visits a hypnotist, only to learn that in a *past* **Life** she was **BLORT**- the Greek Goddess of BOREDOM

PMSAttacks *in literature*

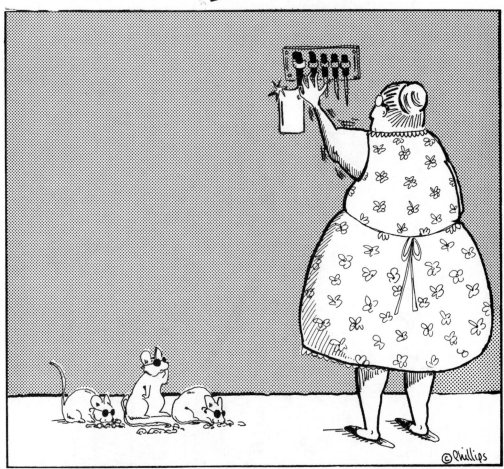

The Three Blind Mice were used to the Farmers Wifes' occasional bursts of anger. **Suddenly**, Stymie senses her reaching for the carving knife

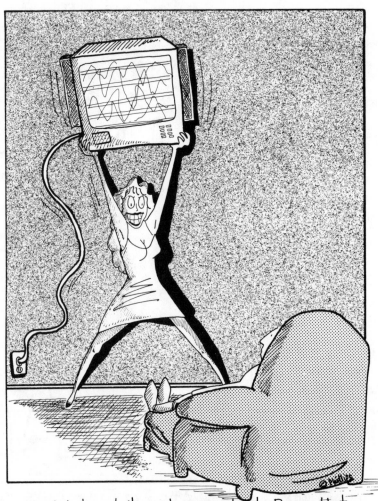

Slowly, but surely, it was becoming clear to Barney that a "PMS Attack" was not the title of an old 1940's grade B-War MOVIE

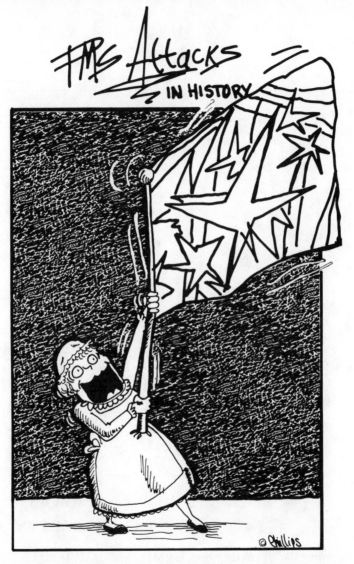

"Betsy ROSS's first attempt at the American Flag"

P.M.S. Attack #25

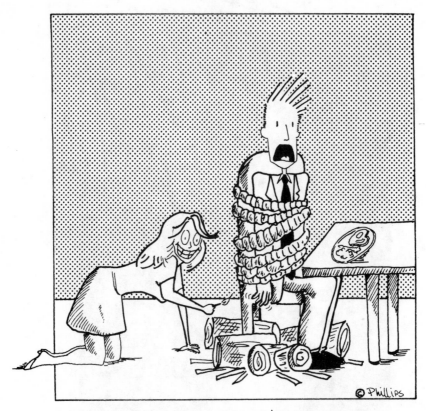

" After breaking up with Barney for
the fourteenth time in one month,
Melinda makes it up to him by
inviting him over for an intimate
candle-light supper. "

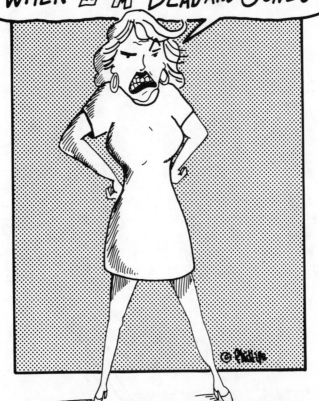

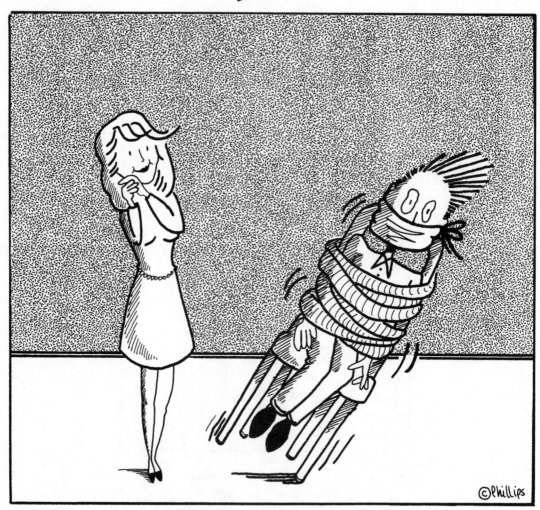

During those times of extreme tension, Melinda enjoyed the company of nice quiet men.

PMS Attacks in History

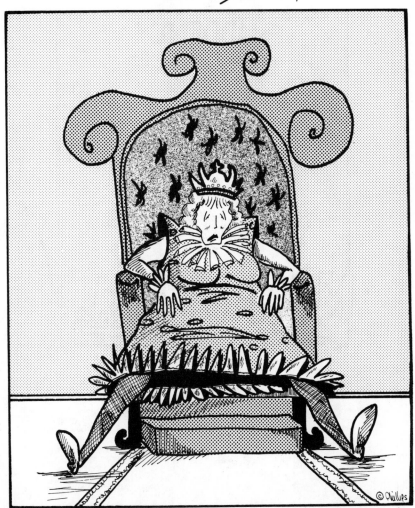

Suffering from severe depression, Catherine the Great
began to feel more like Catherine the Mediocre

P.M.S. Attack #28

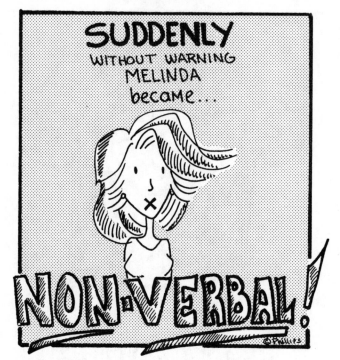

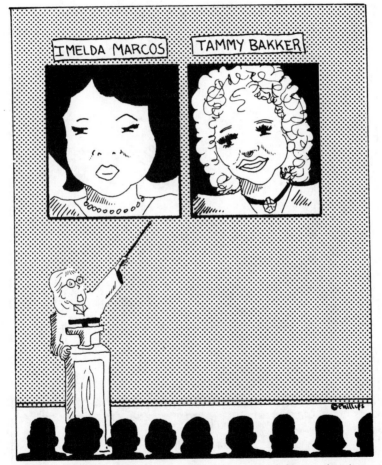

P.M.S. Attack #29

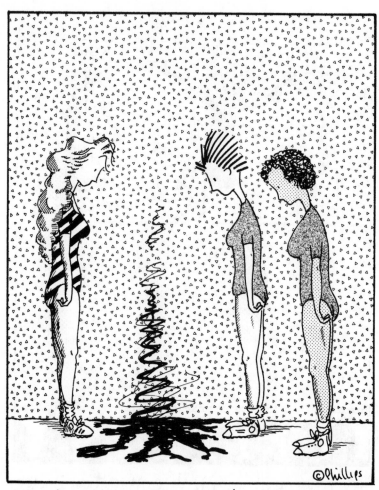

Due to an extreme amount of stress
Melindas friend goes for "the BURN"
for the last time

PMS Attacks

IN HISTORY

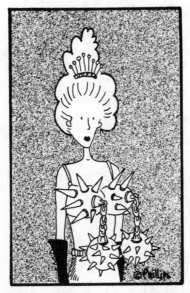

Due to her sensitive breasts,
the Marquis de Sades' wife
found it difficult wearing
her bra

P.M.S. Attack #30

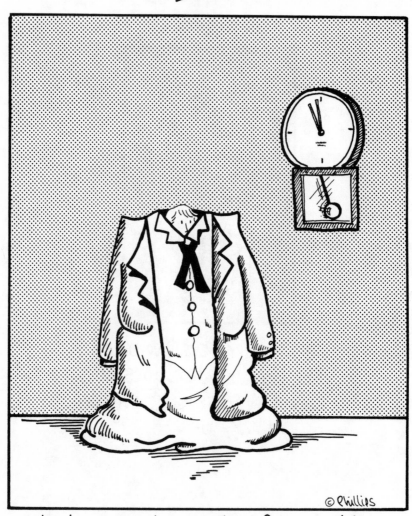

Patiently Melinda waits for another
"FAT ATTACK"

CELEBRITY
PMS Attacks

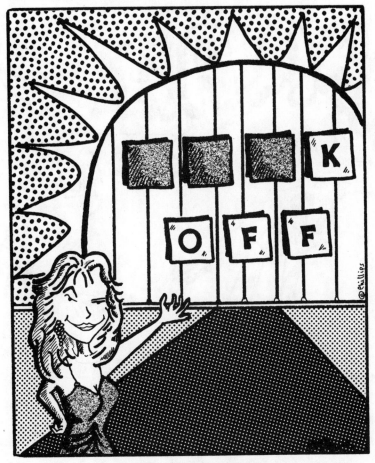

A FAMOUS
GAME SHOW HOSTESS

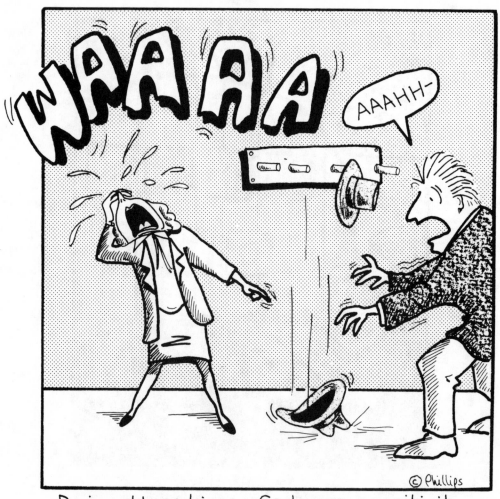

During those times of extreme sensitivity, Melindas' friends knew they had to watch their every move

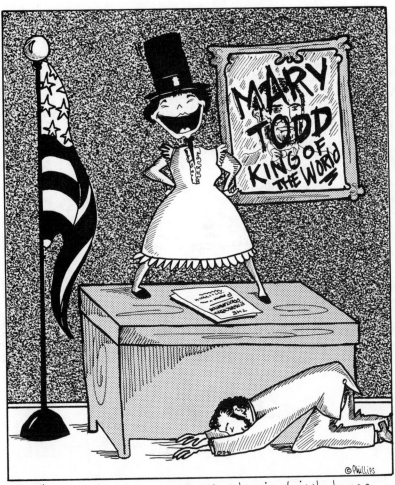

PMS Attacks IN HISTORY

While experiencing a severe chemical imbalance MARY TODD LINCOLN convinces ABE to turn everyone into slaves so that SHE— AND SHE ALONE— could **"RULE THE WORLD!"**

P.M.S. Attack #32

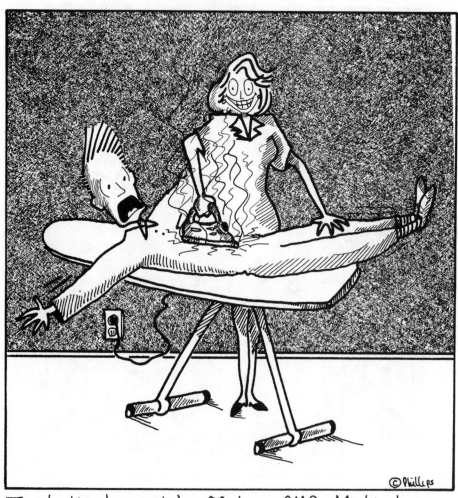

To take her mind off her PMS, Melinda
lovingly irons Barneys shirts

PMS Attacks
in Literature

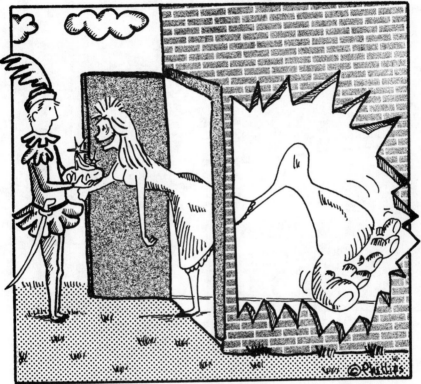

Due to a sudden attack of swollen feet, Cinderella suggests to the Prince that he come back a bit later...
...say in about TWO WEEKS?!!

P.M.S. Attack #33

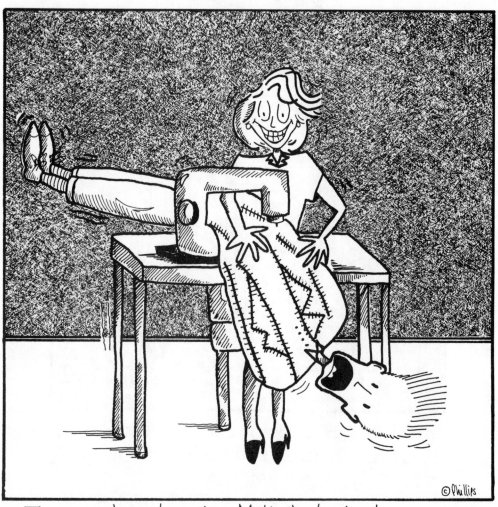

To ease her tension, Melinda lovingly sews
Barney a new suit

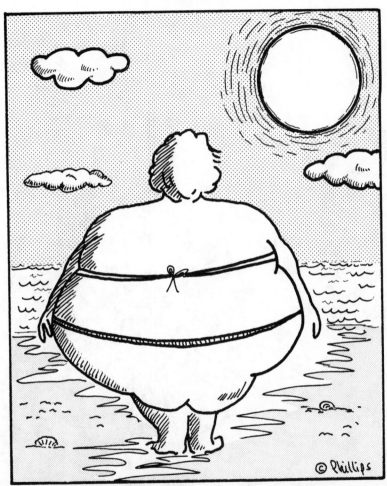

while experiencing severe water
retention, Melinda senses that, in a past
life she was BIMBA, Whale of the Nile

P.M.S. Attack #35

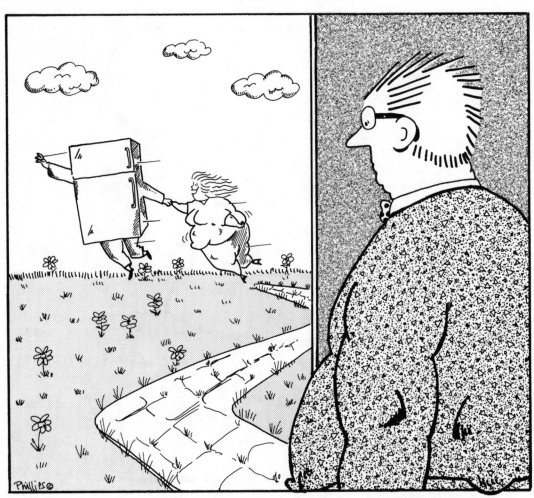

Melinda leaves her Husband and runs away with the refrigerator

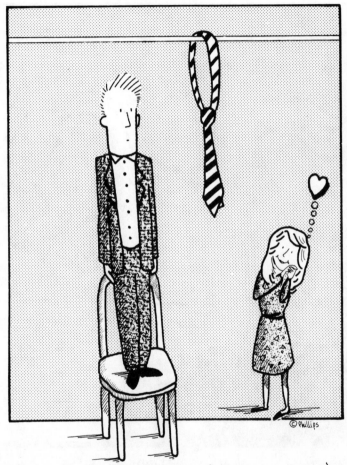

To make up for a recent PMS induced
argument, Melinda buys Barney a new
necktie and waits, with great anticipation,
for him to try it on

P.M.S. Attack #37

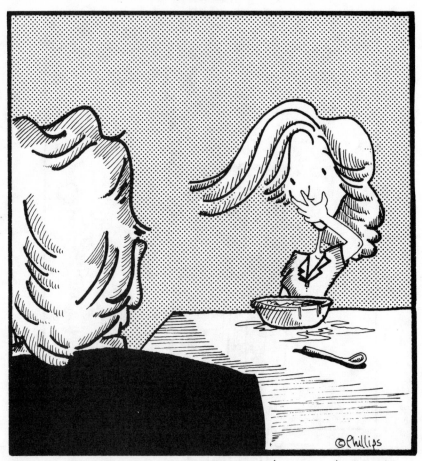

Once again Melinda thought she had it under control. **SUDDENLY**— unbeknownst to Carlos, Melindas' lips fell into the Broccoli soup

PMS Attacks in History

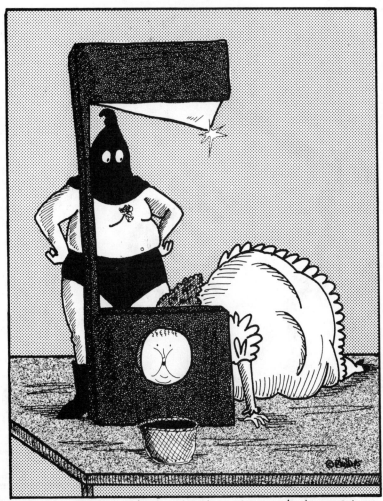

Due to severe water retention, Marie Antoinette was sent to the Guillotine three times before they could fit her face through the hole

P.M.S. Attack #38

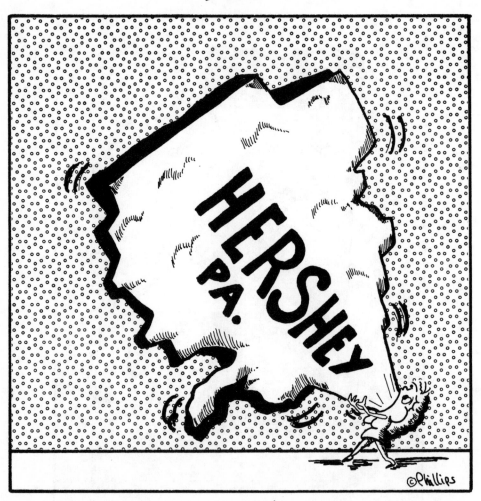

Plaqued by a raging Hormonal imbalance
Melinda devours Hershey, Pennsylvania

AND OTHER INCONVENIENCES OF LIFE

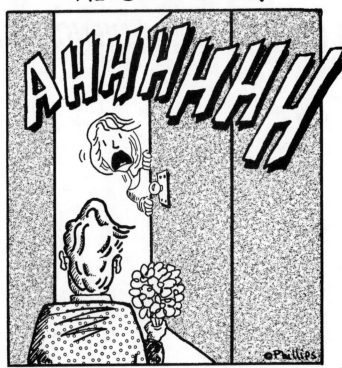

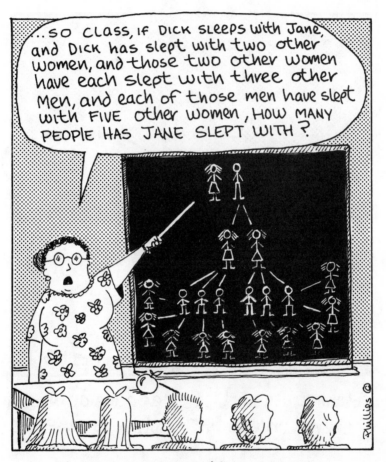

Modern day math problems

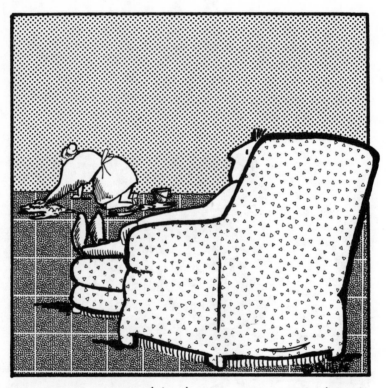

Barney knew that deep inside Angela
there lurked a hot smoldering sex-slave

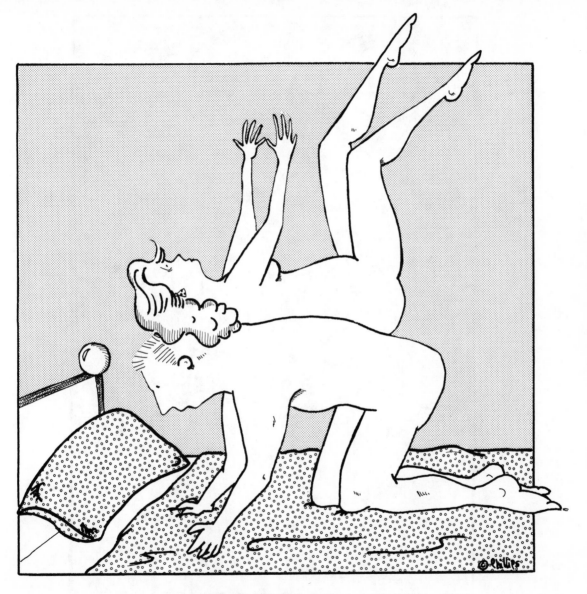

Sufferers of
Sexual Dyslexia

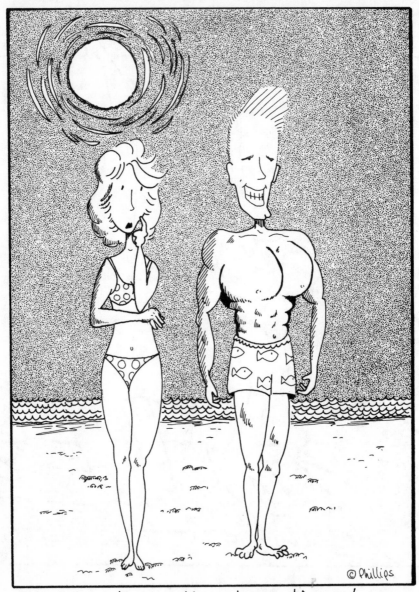

Melinda wonders **whether** she could ever love a
Man whose breasts were bigger than hers

Melinda vowed only to go out
with men who were:
GOOD LOOKING,
           but not self-absorbed
COOL, but caring
SUCCESSFUL, but supportive
FUN, yet responsible

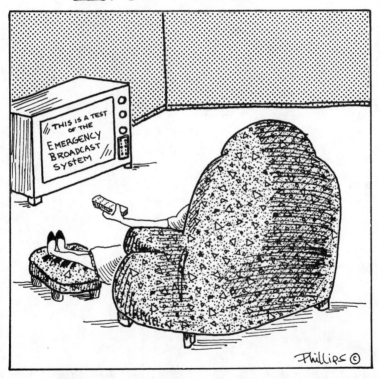

Melinda stayed home a lot.

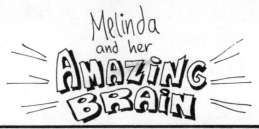

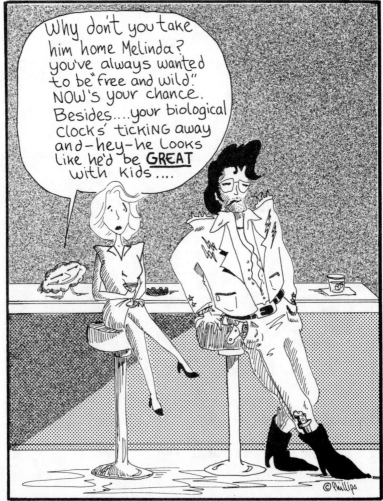

"In a city where the men were either Gay or just plain SLIME, Daphne knew what she had to do...

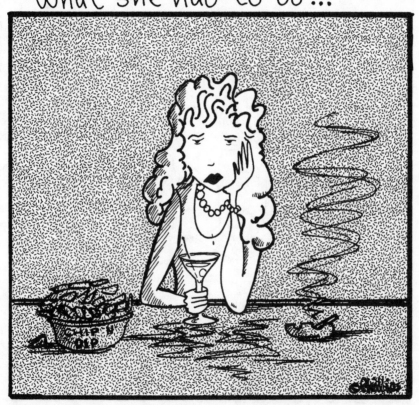

... settle for slime."

Mid-Life Crisis #1

when they were alone it was fine...

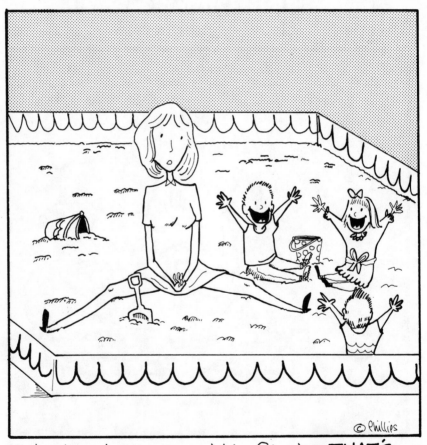

but when she was around his friends—**THAT'S** when Peggy felt she should start dating someone closer to her own age

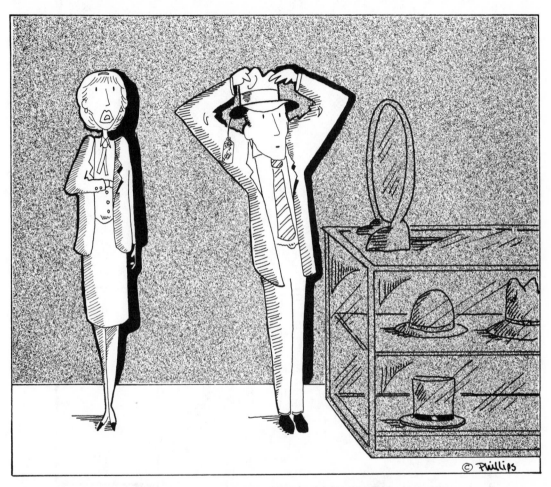

"There he was, the man of my dreams, and **me** without my Business Cards."

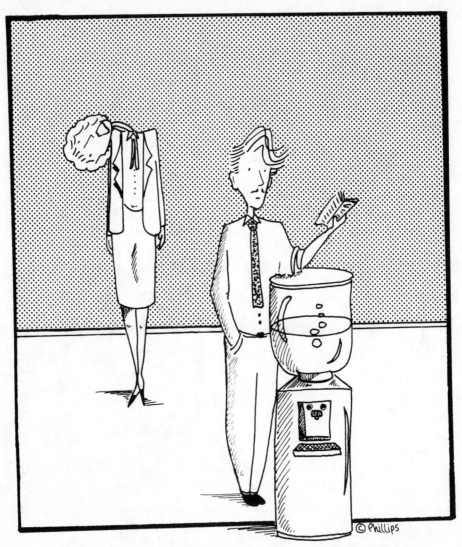

Just when she got the courage to
ask Francois out for a drink, Melindas'
head fell asleep

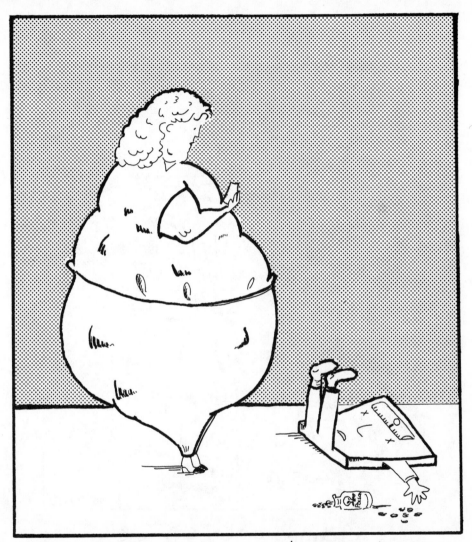

"Upon reading the suicide note left by her scale, Melinda decides to go on a diet."

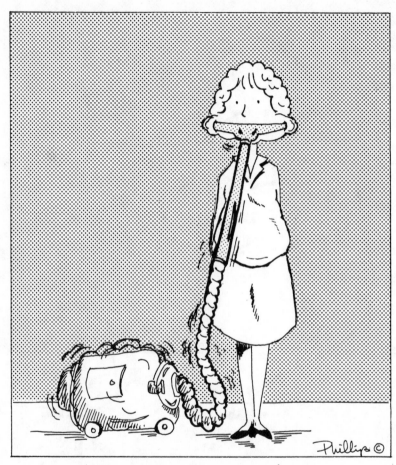

"Melinda goes on the new "Hoover diet.""

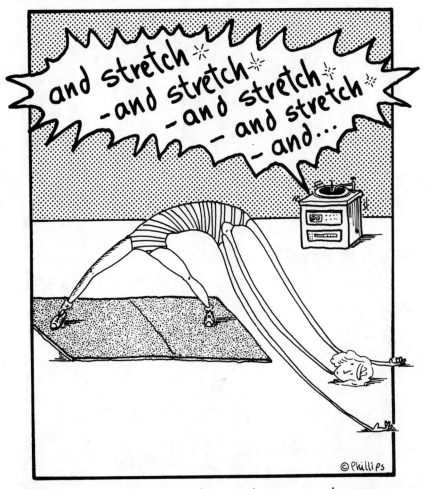

Melinda begins to realize that her
Jane Fonda 'WORKOUT' record has
a skip in it

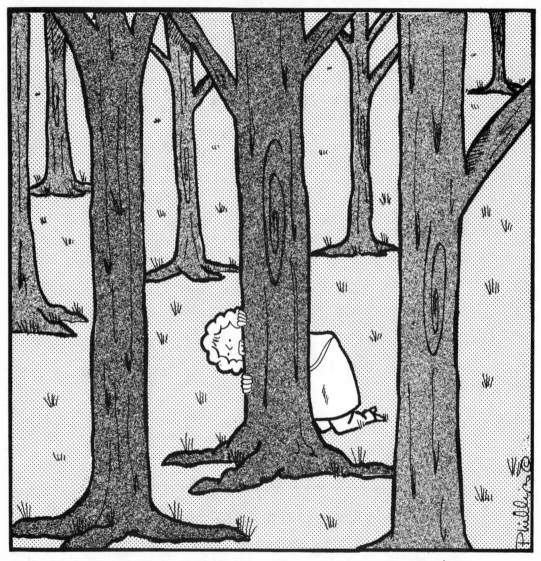

Melinda goes on an all fiber diet

Mid-Life Crisis #2

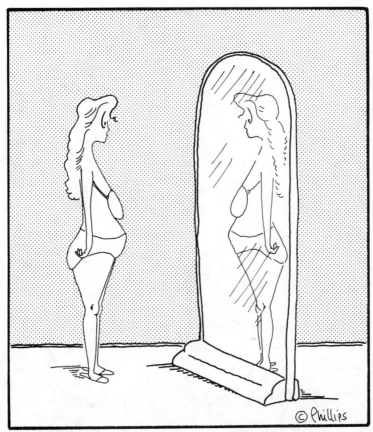

Although she had not yet decided
what she wanted to do with
heR Life, Peggy's body had already
Made up **its** Mind

Mid-Life Crisis #3

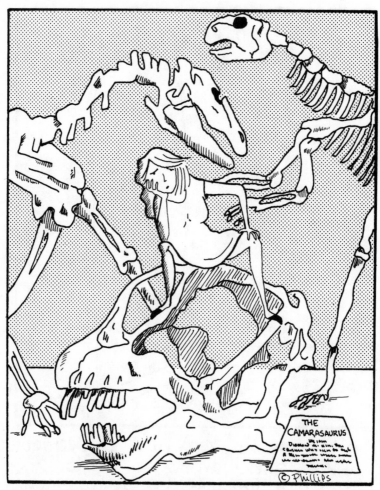

THE CAMARASAURUS

© Phillips

Approaching Mid-life, Peggy found comfort by surrounding herself with things older than she

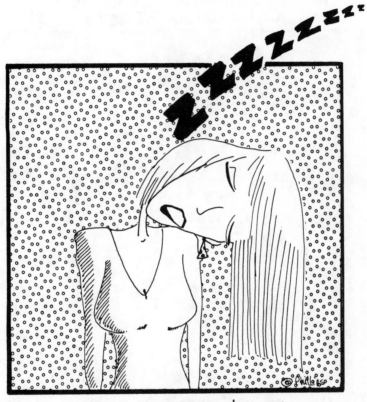

In her quest for "Spiritual enlightenment", Peggy accidently raises her state of unconsciousness

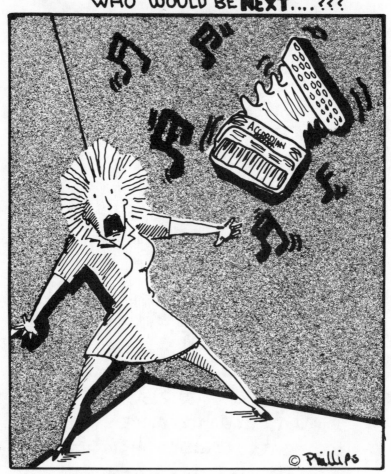

"POLKA-GiEST"

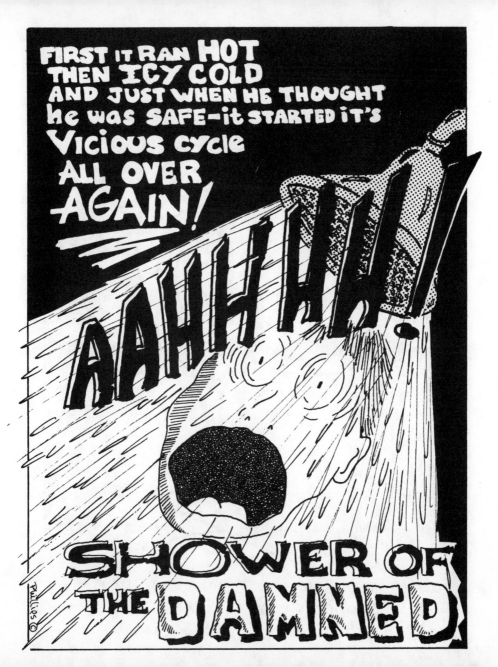

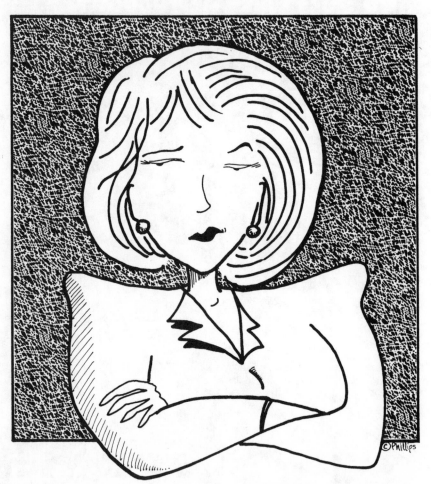

Feeling insecure about her economic future Naomi stopped looking for Mr. Right and started looking for MR. FiLTHY RICH

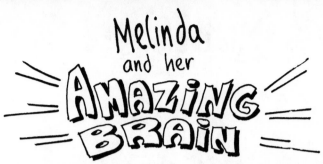

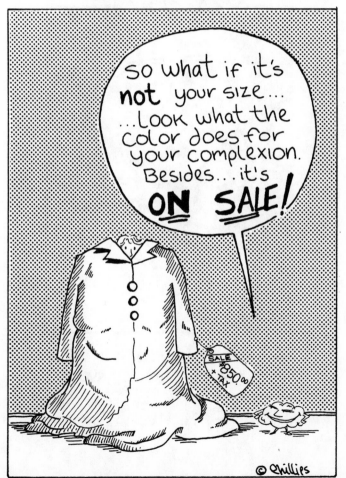

Mid-Life Crisis #5

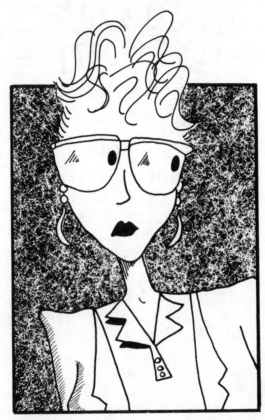

Realizing that she wouldn't stay
young forever, Nadine gave up
Looking for Mr. Right and started
Looking for Mr. Plastic Surgeon

Mid-Life Crisis #6

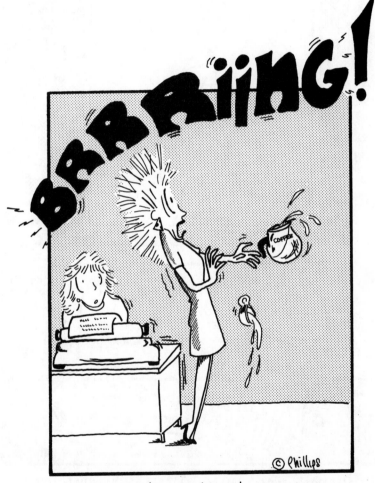

SUDDENLY - without warning -
the alarm on Peggy's BIOLOGICAL CLOCK
went off

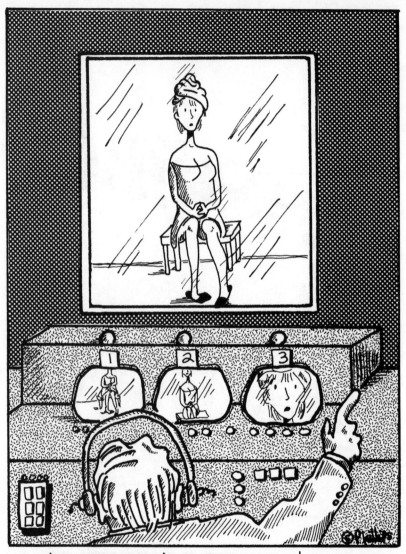

Realizing how damaging suntans are to the skin, Melinda visits Ted Turners' computer colorization Lab

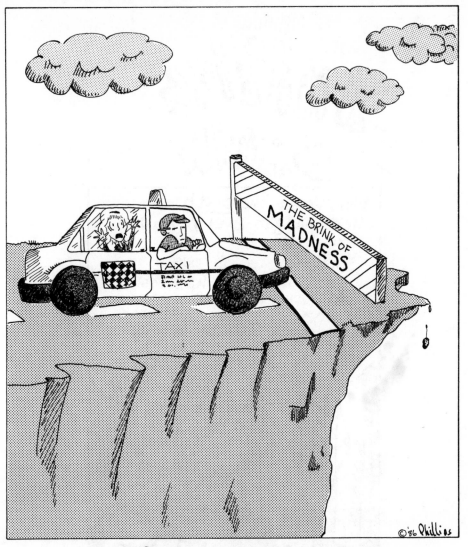

Peggy is driven to
the brink of
Madness

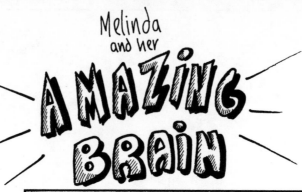

Melinda and her

AMAZING BRAIN

Well, that's the **Sixth** time he's changed **every** word in this letter —

The man is obviously irrational and has lost **ALL** perspective.

why don't you just pick up that typewritter and **THROW it at HIM!**

c'mon Melinda, if **YOU** don't stand up for your rights~**NOBODY** WILL**!!**

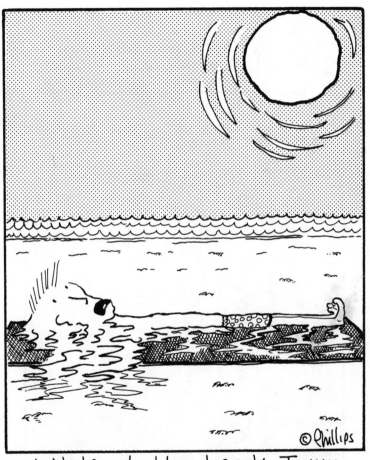

While at the beach Timmy realizes that he forgot to wear his protective sun-screen "timmy realizes he has made a horrible mistake by coming to the Dr. Cyclops EYE Center"

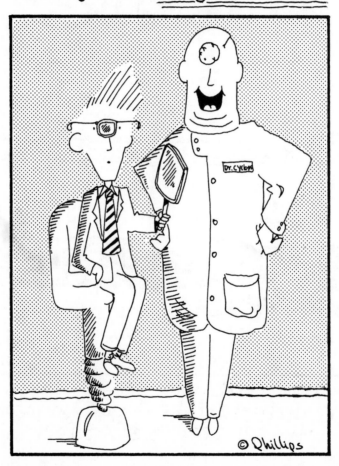

Mid-Life Crisis #7

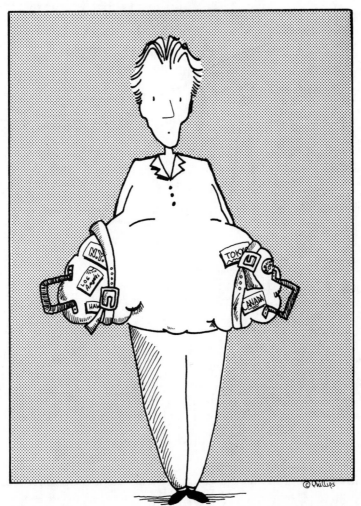

Upon reaching mid-life, Jerrys' "LOVE HANDLES" were now referred to as "Designer Luggage"

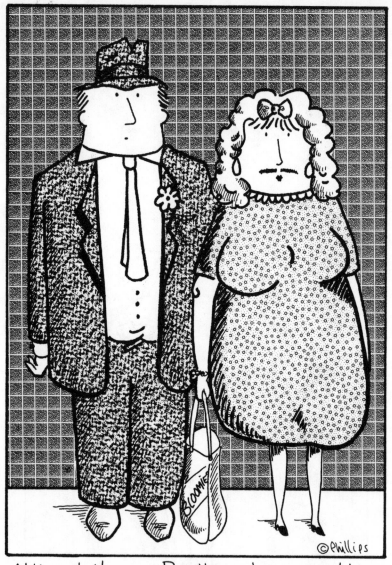

Although it was Bradley who wore the pants in the family, it was Lydia who wore the mustache

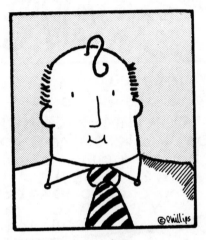

After several months of taking
Minoxidil, Barney is ecstatic that
he can now create the...
" ELVIS LOOK "

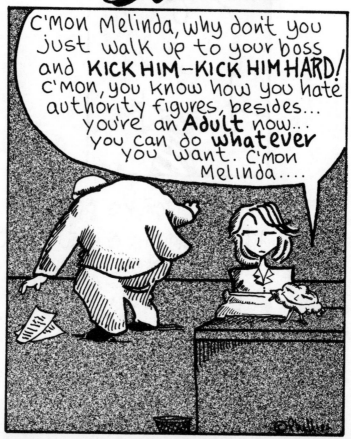

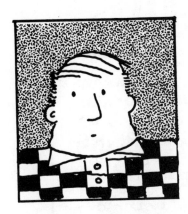

JERRY, BEFORE
USING MINOXIDIL

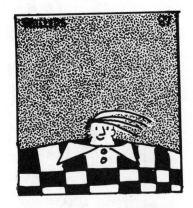

JERRY, AFTER
USING MINOXIDIL—
HIS HEAD NOW
COMPLETELY
COVERED WITH HAIR!

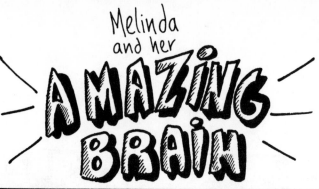

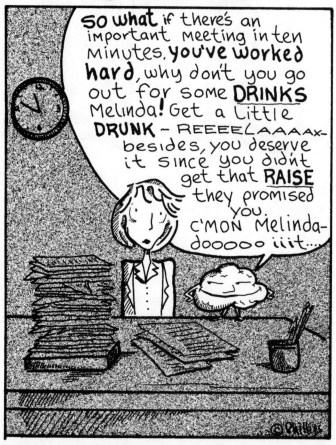

Mid-Life Crisis #8

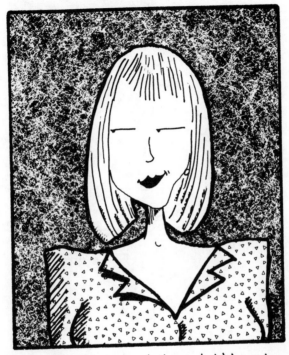

Facing the fact that her child bearing years were coming to an end, Claudia stopped looking for Mr. Right and started looking for Mr. Sperm Bank

NICOTINE Fits: #1

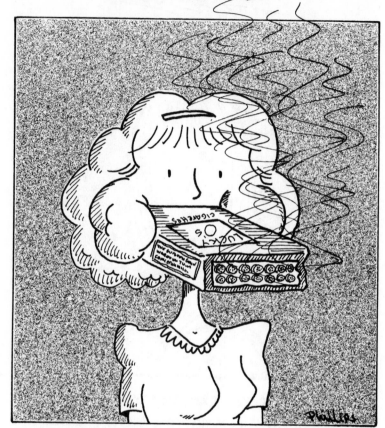

Melinda was determined to cut her smoking down to just one pack a day

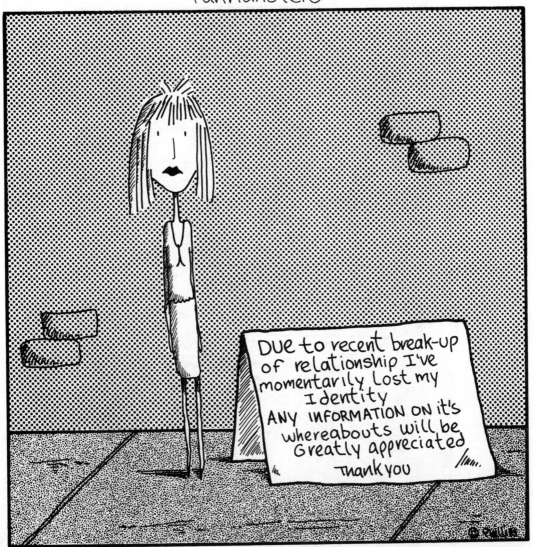

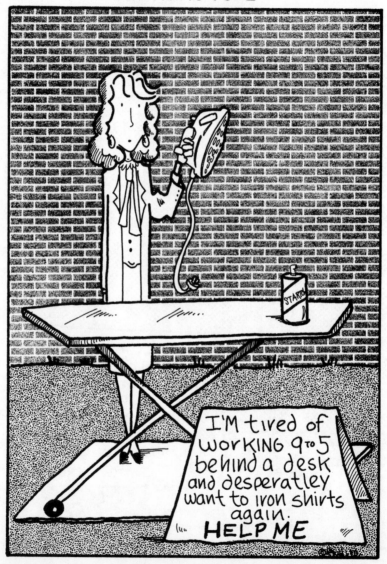

Upwardly Mobile Panhandlers

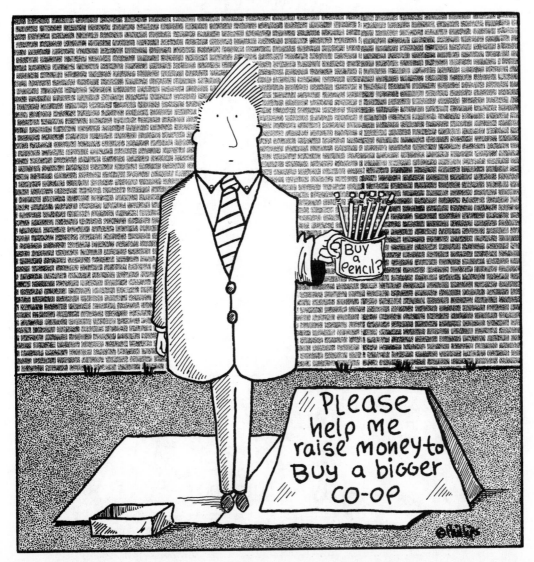

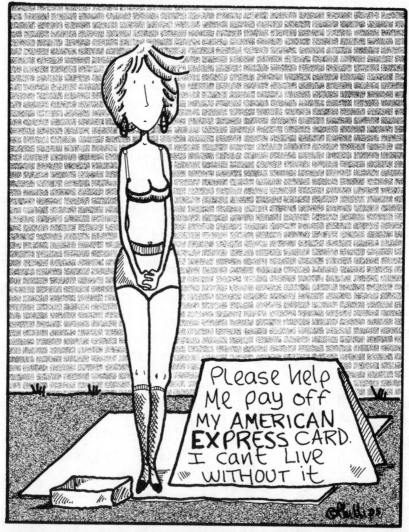

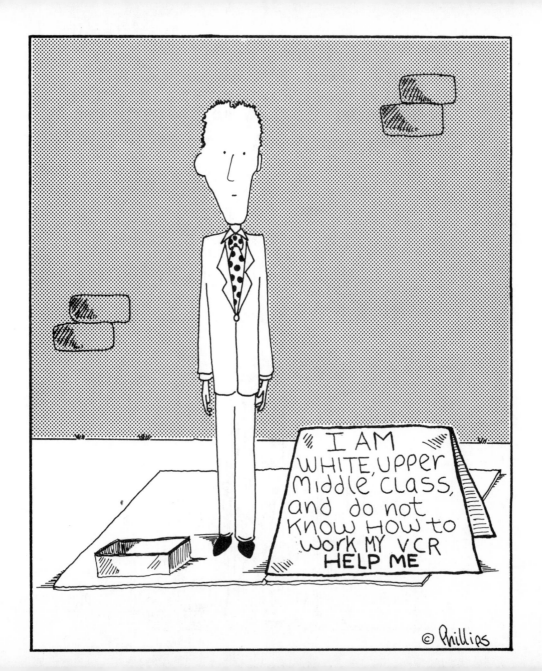

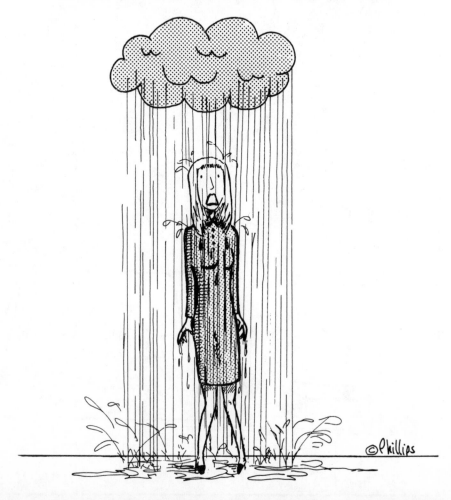

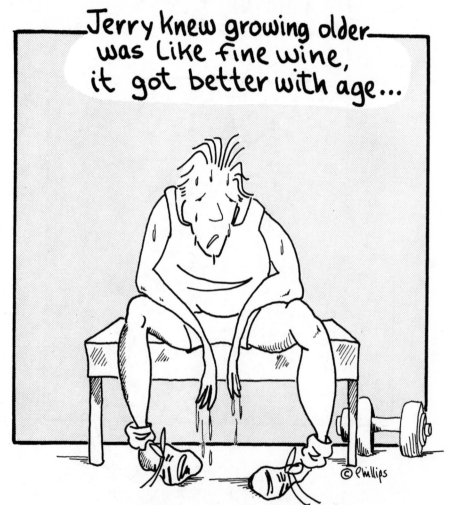

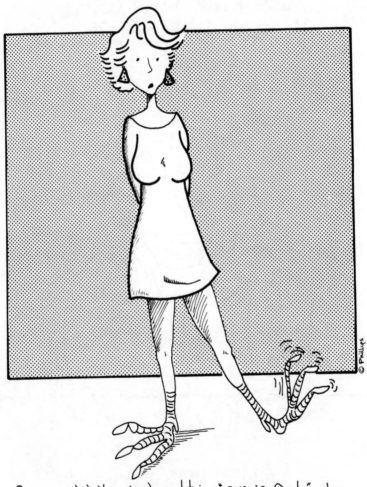

Mid-Life Crisis #9

Peggy didn't mind getting "crows feet", she just never expected them to show up where they did

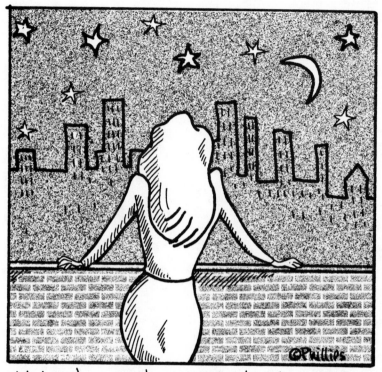

Melinda realizes that all she really wants out of life is... EVERYTHING!